Exhale!

Exhale!

Written by:

Rebecca Boykin

To order additional copies of this book, contact:
Xlibris Corporation
1-888-795-4274
www.Xlibris.com
Orders@Xlibris.com
67364

CONTENTS

ACKNOWLEDGMENTS

I would like to thank all the people in my community. Thank you for your encouragement to complete this book which I call an end time message to the world.

I cannot name everyone; however, the Lord knows who you are.

I salute you and I am honored to know each of you.

I would like to especially highlight and mention those individuals who were directly instrumental in writing and publishing this book:

Dr. Mamie Bryant
Mr. and Mrs. Esley Boykin Jr.
Mr. and Mrs. Larnell D. Boykin
Kamekia N. Victory
Santana Z. Victory
Charles D. Sharon III
Pastors Charles & Josephine Lawton
Evangelist Della Williams
Evangelist Carrie Mae Simon
Tamekia Ford
Last but not least, Professor Gerald Jones

I owe all the praises to the most high, God.

Dear Reader,

I present this book to you to motivate you along the journey called life. Life can be hard at times. One main theme of this book is the saying—No Cross No Crown. You can come out of any situation with the help of the Lord and Savior, Jesus Christ, because I believe that you can do all things through Christ that strengthens you. There is destiny for you and you can reveal your destiny with your hands uplifted and your mouth filled with praise. To God be the glory.

I also desire to see you with a mind to know that this to will pass. You will be ready to go to the next level after reading this publication. Please pass it on to a friend or keep a copy in your personal library. This book will cause a valley situation to become a mountain top experience.

Blessings,
Prophetess Rebecca Boykin

INTRODUCTION

I was inspired to write this book in the midst of some very difficult times. I really felt like I needed to give up, but I heard that a life in Jesus Christ gives you hope. That is when I thought, "I don't have to fight this battle because the battle is not mine it is the Lord's. Immediately thoughts rushed in refreshing me on every level. I think there were times when I did not breathe a full breath. Until the moment I exhaled!

Great motivation surged, inspiration kicked in, and faith pulled me through. I had gone through so much until it will take even more writing to tell you how I made it over unharmed.

I give God the praise. You can also do this. Just read each word carefully about our immutable God. Apply this word and your spirit will become lifted and you will become illuminated with a mind to trust God. You will be educated and soon you will be able to declare; it is over now.
Hallelujah!

Exhale for the Lord our God is with you!

PREFACE

Serving under pressure can be a hindrance in your life whether spiritual or just living in this world. To keep a sound mind we need a supernatural experience to EXHALE. In the natural what do we do? We release out a breath of fresh air that helps us function properly and feel better.

Whoever is reading this book whether it be two' o'clock in the morning or wherever you are. You are about to receive a miracle. I believe everything happens through divine appointment. You may be going through something that has held you captive for too long. Our biggest problem is that we don't really know how to let go. Life changes have boxed us in since childhood. Trials have branded us.

Show me your ways, O Lord, teach me your paths, guide me in
your truth and teach me, for you are God my savior, and
my hope is in you all day long—Psalm 25: 4&5

STAND STILL

We don't do so good rushing or running. Exhaling pressure comes off at ease. Listen to the voice as God speaks to you through these messages as I write a fresh anointing is on these pages to help you realize that you can come through whatever faces you today. This is due to the fact God has chosen to be a help to His people around the world. We can be in a certain place, but we can write and let books be placed far and near. So take another exhale about now and let the Holy Spirit do what only He can do for your life today.

If it had not been for a moment in this present life with God on our side ; some of us would have gone off the deep edge. Let me tell you a little bit about the deep edge through my personal testimonies. I'll help you out by sharing a few of them. From childhood I was raised by my matriarchal grandmother, a beautiful woman, affectionately known as "Grandma Lizzie". Her proper name was Lizzie Jones. Grandma Lizzie was a tall, bronze skinned woman with high cheek bones. Of course we believe she was of Native American descent. Grandma was a strict disciplinarian. She raised me with tough love. Life was sometimes a struggle. I was reared in a small unincorporated town called Orange Mills, Florida. Maybe you never heard of Orange Mills. Orange Mills is located approximately five miles east of Palatka, Florida. Well if you haven't heard of Palatka, Florida; it lies approximately fifty miles south of Jacksonville, Florida. Orange mills is so small that we don't have a traffic light. The biggest thing in Orange Mills is the four lane highway that runs through. Grandma Lizzie and I shared a home in Orange Mills. At time this small wooden house was occupied by Me, my grandmother and numerous family members. We survived due to our strong family structure. Family was a top priority to my grandmother. Grandma Lizzie went home to be with the Lord many years ago. I continue to reside in Orange Mills. I loved Grandma Lizzie very dearly. When she

passes away I was grief stricken, but I had to let go. This was my first trial
of the deep edge

As I think back, I remember Grandma Lizzie becoming ill. I had to
be there for her when she got to the point that she couldn't do things for
herself. I was surely glad to be there. However being the eldest girl in the
house; I was a loner. Back in those days elderly people did not play with a
twig off of a tree or a belt. They would whip your back side and tell you to
shut up right now. I felt left out, but don't get me wrong, the chastisement
did help in some way. Somewhere through that part in my life I felt shut in
and did not know how to release out. I loved the good part, but still I felt
captured. Through school I knew I was cared for but something just wasn't
right. This is what I thought within.

My mother and stepfather were migrant workers. I would see them go
away every summer. They would go north to harvest crops in Virginia. If I
could have explained how I felt, I probably could have let go and exhaled
then, but I couldn't. So I held on to it. I hope that you will be blessed as
you read through these chapters the many testimonies of God's goodness.

The supernatural will work for us if we just listen. Listen to me; our
problems are nothing for God. We must take one day at a time. This is
easier said than done. You have tried everything and everything has failed.
Now try Jesus. We have got to get a grip.

GET A GRIP

We need a plea for guidance like the psalmist David. We need the Lord to help our mind. The mind is the devil's playground. Until we get a grip we need to ask for understanding; like I am; you're so old, but the beginning is to realize that we need to ask the Lord for wisdom. I feel so good writing my first book, and I pray that the anointing on this book will lift you out of whatever you are experiencing.

> *33 Teach me, O Lord, to follow your decrees. 34 Give me understanding and I will keep your law and obey it with all my heart. 35 Direct me in the path of your command. 36 Turn my heart toward your statutes and not towards selfish gain. 37 Turn my eyes away from worthless things preserve my life according to your word.38 Fulfill your promise to your servant, So that you may be feared. 39 Take away the disgrace I dread, for your laws are good. 40 How I long for your precepts! Preserve my life in your righteousness. Psalm 119: 33-40*

> *Right about here, dear friend, I would like to pause and pray*
> *that your anchor will hold and grip the solid rock;*
> *that rock is Jesus. He is the one.*
> *Our father we realize that we all have sinned and come short of*
> *your glory, but I ask you to stretch out your mighty hand*
> *and heal, deliver and set free in Jesus' name. Amen*

I feel an experience from heaven overshadowing as I continue to write. When a person gets a grip it is for some significant reason. Believe me, if a man is drowning and he is able to make it to a floating tree branch; He will hold onto that branch for dear life. Life can be so uncertain. A shift can bring changes. It could be an unexpected divorce, sickness, lack of money for bills. I can tell you about life changes because I have been there and done that. So get a grip and keep persevering.

So you did go off the deep edge. I see you have a chance. You may ask yourself; how does she know? If you are holding this book in your hands keep reading. I asked God how I can get the word to your people, a prophetic word to heal and deliver. He said "Write it".

Just before the birth of my second son I experienced a deep edge situation. I had to get a grip. When things began to settle down; I mean from pill popping, because there are time you just can't handle if you don't get the right care, meaning medical attention. So, don't feel like you are a super star. It is the Lord our God who gave the doctors knowledge to help. I sought medical doctors to help me. One day I thought about the mighty power of God and believed God's word. I told myself I am going to walk through this with the word of God and a special friend in my life. This woman is a woman of wisdom, Dr. Mamie Bryant. She is my pastor and mentor. I walked through it and almost twenty-eight years later I continue to walk.

When we are of the world we will get upset if someone hurts us. We will say I am going to get you back. Well let's turn this thing around; it was Satan that brought this attack on your life. You're walking in the word.

Take the helmet of salvation and the sword of the Spirit,
which is the Word of God.
Ephesians 6:17

Christians need to speak the words; these words come out of the mouth of Jesus. So we can speak it out of our own mouth and subdue the work of the enemy. God's word is powerful.

For the Word of God is living and active; sharper than any two
edged sword. It penetrates even to dividing soul and spirit, joint
and marrow, It judges the thoughts and attitudes of the heart.
Hebrews 4:12

I have given you a few testimonies just to encourage you to go to the next level. Do not dwell on things of the past. Let it go. Exhale and know that Jesus cares for you. I practically live by Psalm 91:11-

For he shall give his angels charge over thee, to keep thee in all thy ways

In other words the Lord orders his angels to protect us wherever we go. Sometimes we just see through the darkness, which seems to be drifting in on us. You must learn in this time of darkness to trust God even when you can't hear him speak to you. God's timing is so much different from our timing. We want to know direction. We want things to happen quickly, but it doesn't always work like that. As we learn how to wait on God, God is faithful and true to his promises. The things he has promised, He is well able to perform. He has promised to be with us always. He is a comforter and keeper in all situations. This should make us persevere until his time of illumination comes.

Believe me, when the Lord illuminates or brings light to the situation He will bring joy unspeakable joy. The best thing about it is this allows us to have joy in tribulation because we are not just walking along. We are walking in the Word of God.

It is giving me great pleasure to write this book which is long past due. When we don't obey God, We put our souls at risk. We can think straight because we hear the Lord speaking to us daily concerning our walk with him. So, I am happy to journey through with this book. I believe others will come naturally if I obey.

BE PATIENT

Being patient can be one of the hardest tasks in your life. Circumstances in our life will teach us how to be patient. Here are some hints for our health. I found that anxiety is a desperate situation. There are things we cannot change. Yet we want to change them so badly. We try as hard as we can to fix it on our own until we lose sleep for days and make ourselves sick. But, when you understand how important it is to wait; it is worthwhile.

> *That ye be not slothful, but followers of them who through faith*
> *and patience inherit the promises.*
> *Hebrews 6:12*

We never know the tool that is used for the kingdom. Serving patiently is a wonderful tool which is a witness to others. I believe it will get stronger and stronger over our lives. On the journey walking our walk will determine how we get there and when we get there. Out of all the preaching and prophesying we have nobody can exhale for us. Make up in our mind to practice patience. A mentor will help, one that you can listen to. No matter how tough they sound; when they instruct us sometimes it sounds like a noise in our ear, but hang tough. We need each other, but again I say nobody can exhale for you. Some deep situation has almost knocked us to our knees, but about now this is where we need to take some time out and kneel in the presence of our Lord and Savior. A lot of times we did not realize He was there all the time, but there comes a time we can see the break of day. Your day break is coming thru. I hope that you are being rejuvenated and receiving a lot more strength.

I am going to prophesy over your life. I pray that this will take you to the next level. For the Lord our God sees you and He knows where you are. My child, you may be on a bus or a plane, and yet I know where you are in this situation. So rise and go forward because I am the Lord thy God. I am with thee. Rejoice!

A WORD OF ENDURANCE

Since you have purified your souls in obeying the truth, through the spirit in sincere love of the brethren love one another fervently with a pure heart. Acts 15:9

An enduring word can change the way we think or feel. There are many circumstances which we cannot change, but change can take place through the Spirit by sincere love for the brethren. Let us love one another with a pure heart. As amazing as it sounds we are stunned to the move of the Spirit through the word of God. We can go through the valley of decisions with direction. I have found that there can be peace in the midst of a storm. We can ask the Lord to help us look up to you in the midst of a storm.

We can press toward the mark and then all that we confront makes us light up with joy. Because we believe that the joy of the Lord is our strength. Strength is what we need to confront the forces that are in this present world. We are bound to go through some stuff. God knows where we are right now. God will protect us from temptation. He always gives us a way to avoid falling into the enemies' hand.

So surely, with such a love protecting you rejoice. Be content the Lord is with you (Hebrews 13:5) Mighty God; I rejoice that you will never forsake me!

A lamp unto my feet

When we exhale I believe our whole body lights up. The Earth lights up from the Sun and Moon. Send us light. Safe in the hands of God we find a path that is revealed by the light of the Word of God. When the light shined about Peter when he was imprisoned it manifested that Christ himself is a lamp and a light. The Lord our God will be a light to you also. All you have to do is ask.

I want to stop here and ask the Lord to be that light and lamp:

> *Dear Lord,*
>   *As this reader walks through the word in these pages; I ask you,*
> *in the name of Jesus, Order the steps of your people and Dear Lord,*
> *Light their path, and be a lamp unto their feet.*

God's word is a precious gift to us. We can appreciate it because the word contains the truth and direction we need to live a godly life. Overcoming fear, we need to use our faith over fear.

> *Confront fear head on 2 Timothy 1:7*

God has not given us a spirit of fear, but of power and love and of a sound mind. There is some good fear, fear that alerts us in the time of danger. It gives us time to avoid some of the dangerous situations. Then we can exhale and tell the Lord thank you. Never let Satan sound like a lion roaring in your ears.

> *So be sober, be vigilant; because your adversary the devil walks*
> *about like a roaring lion, seeking whom he may devour. Resist him,*
> *steadfast in faith, know that the same suffering are experienced by*
> *your brotherhood in the world Peter 5:89*

Fear is a stubborn phenomenon. It will not just go away, but when we trust God, knowing that God has not given us the spirit of fear, but power to boldly confront your fear and bring down the walls that have held you captive.

The lion roars to make known that he is king of the jungle, but in this case see what the word of God says about it. It says Satan roars like a lion; so when Satan roars confront that fear by faith; meet him at your heart's door, when he knocks send faith to answer.

> *For a great and effective door has been opened to me and there are*
> *many adversaries. 1 Corinthians 16:9*

The best way to overcome the devil and his demons is to stay in God's will and when you are in His will He will protect us. I have been under Dr. Mamie Bryant as a pastor for many years. I believe she is called after God's own heart. I have seen the church go through some real sticky crises, and she will say lets stand against that Satan is trying to do. I want to say to you, Christian friend, stand strong against the adversary. If you keep pressing and trusting in the leadership of the Holy Spirit you will find out this one roaring like a lion doesn't even have teeth. You will come out unharmed—Give the Lord praise!

I find it to be a true fact that if you are doing anything for God the enemy will attack you. When you think about not spending you life struggling against the devil to serve God; you stand strong in the authority given to you by Jesus. Greater is He who is in you that he who is in the world. See 1 John 4:4

Set some goals in life and don't give up. Say within yourself—I refuse to lose. I had a golden opportunity to raise three wonderful grandchildren along with my two boys, Esley Jr. and Larnell D. Boykin. Charles made it to the NFL. Kamekia is Pharmacy Tech. Both girls served in the U.S. Army. Santana works for Georgia Pacific in Palatka FL.

REFUSE TO LOSE

The odds were against us. Their mom has been incarcerated for about seven years for manslaughter, problems at an early age, but I love her so much until I had to get a grip. Walk in the word and all of the greatness that can keep you alive and well. I got angry with Satan and said I refuse to lose here. You might well get back! I am going after what I see. I see children needing to be developed into men and women. They need to get to college and go to work. By the way Esley is a Special education teacher. He loves it. Larnell works at the local Youth Academy in Hasting Fl, the Potato Capital, and a city you might want to visit sometime.

Getting back to basics; Behold the Lord thy God has set the land before thee. Go up and posses it, as the Lord God of thy fathers has said unto thee: fear not. Neither be discouraged. Deuteronomy 1:21

Sometime we are all faced with disappointments and failure in life. Plans that fail, but you must make a decision and adapt and adjust. You must approach a new season of this situation. Keep going despite your feeling. Every time you are confronted think of the greater one inside of you. When setbacks would come I would rise above discouragement through Him who lives in me. That is what you have to do; rise about and know Jesus live through you. All of my boys earned football scholarships. My living room looks like a trophy room. To God be the glory for the things He has done. Don't stop. Refuse to lose. Go to your destiny. There is a place just waiting for you. Whether you are on your way to college or you may already be retired. You need a life. Refuse to lose. Trust in what God has in store. Because what God has for you it is for you.

You must be covered, like a good friend might say I got you back. This means they are watching. What you can't see you must wear God's armor and stand your ground. This is the way if you are going to resist the devil and go to a level and do all God wants you to do. You can't have your way. Be led by the leading of the Holy Spirit. The shield of faith, lift it up and stand your ground.

> *Therefore put on God's complete armor, that you may be able to resist and stand your ground on the evil day and, having done all to stand; stand therefore. Ephesians 6:13*

The armor is a perfect example of a soldier being covered with protective helmet, breastplate and shield. You learn of God's keeping power. Know he is with us. Your mind is made up and your heart is fixed. No matter how much pressure is on you. You are on your way. Just trust God.

> *Being confident of this very thing, that He who has begun a good work in you will complete it until the day of Jesus Christ. Philippians 1:6*

O give thanks unto the Lord for He is good. If you had not prayed a trust his far the devil would already have overwhelmed you. But you are overwhelmed daily about what God can do. You daily life can have a retreat in the presence of the lord. You need a place of refuge. So our God is a rock of Salvation.

> *In you, O Lord, I put my trust. Let me never be put to shame. Deliver me in your righteousness and cause me to escape. Incline your ear to me and save me. Be my strong refuge to which I may resort continually. You have been the commandment to save me. For you are my rock and my fortress. Psalm 71*

Never fail to ask for help. If you give to the Lord He will take it. The Lord says this to you: Be not afraid or dismayed all this great multitude; for the battle is not yours, but God's 2 Chronicles 20:15

You may not know how to stand against such great army of sickness, army of bills, you name it, but you can do like Jehosophat, King of Judah. Lord will you exercise judgment upon them? You don't know what to do but keep your eyes on the Lord. He will fix it.

We do not realize that the Lord is right beside us. Trust and obey. Never try to carry such a heavy load. As I sense, hear, this whole book is about the love of God coming to our rescue. I heard a friend say; when I call the Lord He will come to my rescue. You can save time and worry. So rise up Christian friend and realize which side you're on. Stand up if you are on the winning side. As you walk closer to God you are covered with a covering Satan himself can't touch. You will come through this. Your maker, which is God, has called you into a righteous life and as you walk keep your head up.

I prophesy to you right now that no weapon formed against thee shall prosper. You are blessed and wherever your feet trod as you walk with me saith thou God even the ground will be blessed.

SOWING SEEDS

Whatsoever a man soweth, that shall he also reap. Galatians 6:7

As children of God, I believe we are here on Earth with a purpose. I feel like that purpose is to do right and glorify God. So many times instead we are up tight and in our own world. But when you do right you bring glory to God. You bring glory by telling others of his goodness. This is manifesting his excellence in a beautiful way. You can bring a blessing to others in many ways. You build them up by compliment. Sometimes express a pat on the back or thank you to encourage them along the way.

So you see we can get busy. We don't always have money to help one another, but sow and show some love. If someone offends you; Exhale. Forgive them! I encourage you to treat everybody with love and respect. You will be glorifying God and also receiving your blessing by reaping what you sow God gets the glory. Put your trust in Jesus—Psalm 23:1

The Lord is my Sheppard. I shall not want. He maketh me to lie down in green pastures. He leads me beside the still waters. He restores my soul. He leads me in the path of righteousness for his name sake. Yea though I walk through the valley of the shadow of death I will fear no evil. For you are with me. Your rod and your staff, they comfort me. You prepare a table before me in the presence of my enemies. You anoint my head with oil. My cup runneth over. Surely goodness and mercy shall follow me all the days of my life and I will dwell in the house of the Lord forever.

Just as the Lord was a Sheppard for David he can be your leader. Everyone can share from this act of love. Business, spiritual, political leaders should realize that Jehovah is their Sheppard. David was a keeper of the sheep, but the Lord was the keeper of David.

A prayer of trust and faith

Our father we recognize how great you are and I thank you for this day that you have allowed us to see. I am trusting in your holy hand; that when I am touched I will believe and receive by your power in Jesus name. Amen.

One should never worry when you pray, because if you pray then don't worry. And if you worry don't pray. Put your trust in God. Why worry?

Cease from anger and forsake wrath; fret not yourself—Psalm 37:8

Anxiety is an attack that can work to destroy you mind. I escaped more devastation than I can tell you: depression, stress, and everything attacks. They follow one after the other, but you don't have to go that route. Stop and take charge. These attacks come to keep you from serving the Lord. Satan uses the tools for his weapons to press your faith down. So you cannot be victorious, but don't you be pressed. Worry is something you may not realize is there. You may call it something else, but it is still worry.

I want to tell you here to cast all your cares on the Lord, because the Lord cares for you. He knows what you are going through. Many of us never take a second thought about getting in our beds at night. We have complete confidence that our beds are capable of providing us with a comfortable night sleep. We don't worry about the bed holding us. Sometimes we probably just roll over. Just roll over on God. We can have full confidence in Him. We can also have divine rest in the Lord.

Hasten to Obey

You need a wall against procrastination. Are you the director of your department? Are you contemplating organizing a bible school? Procrastination is one of the tactics Satan uses to keep you away from God. When you make plans to do what God wants do not listen to Satan. So don't put off today, say you will do this tomorrow. Obedience to God is not something you do in your spare time. It should be the number one priority on your agenda. Do it now. God give me the strength to pursue your purpose for my life.

Help

Pride will set you up for a great fall. You don't know what to do when Satan attacks. Everything we accomplish is done with the help and blessing of God. When Satan attacks you through persecution, physical condition, like sickness, the best solution is complete obedience to the word. In the word you will find a hiding place. You need to dwell in the secret place of the almighty God (Psalm 91:1)

Ask God to defend you against the attacks of Satan. You need to turn to God and ask for help. Right about here exhale for the Lord your God is with you. To abide under the shadow of the almighty God. You must get in that place so when the attacks come you are already covered.

When you are attacked forgive your attackers. Pray for them, by doing this you are responding with obedience to God. Father I put my trust in you, and I will cry out for help in a needy time.

Rejoice and exalt in hope. Be steadfast and patient in suffering and tribulations, be constant in prayer.

Romans 12:12

Be so constant in prayer until you will have a prayer of mercy and at the same time you need to meditate on how excellent the Lord is. David asked the Lord and so can you. Bow down your ear O Lord, hear me for I am poor and needy. Preserve my life, for I am holy. You are my God. Save you servant who trusts in you! Be merciful to me O Lord for I cry to you all day long. Rejoice the soul of your servant for to you, O Lord, I lift up my soul for you, Lord are good, and ready to forgive and abundant in mercy to all those who call upon you.

I came from a poor family, but we had a lot of love in our home. I was also raised by an uncle. His name was James Sinclair Jones Sr. We called him Uncle Bubba. He was a man of courage. My uncle fought a fight with cancer some years ago. He never neglected to pray. I never questioned God why I just appreciated the years he let Uncle Bubba live in the midst of the family in a little town called Orange Mills, FL

You can cry out to God for help. The Jones family did. The Lord will hear your cry. So keep your eyes on the word. This verse deals with your faith, just think about it if you needed a favor from mom or dad, or even your boss. Are you likely to get that favor if you have been doing a messy job? Maybe you did not do your chores at home like you should have. Would you even ask if your work was a mess? When you follow the directions of God you will have more confidence to ask the Lord for help whenever you need it.

Many years ago I was sick unto death. A friend told me all the works you have done and lived and life holiness, you have conducted yourself upright before God, and she said you can remind Him at that time. I was not a bible scholar, had not studied too much. But I believe what she said, and then I appealed to God for my deliverance from the spirit of oppression. The Lord did it for me.

You too can be delivered from under attacks that have been from side to side. Cling to faith in God's word. There is great comfort, protection and deliverance which can be found in Psalm 119-121.

Let's pray right here: Lord this day, I am going to study your word, because I believe this is our only sure source of comfort. Amen.

Be of good courage for your help is much nearer that you realize, you have wasted so much time, just living a life. Well it's time for you to live a life that the Lord has for you. Abundance is just abundance and I read in the word where the Lord says I come that you may have life and have it more abundantly.

We can have what we say, you need to open your mouth and speak positive; believing you can have what you say. God's help is for those who seek him. Just lift up your eyes to the hills. I will lift up my eyes to the hills from whence comes my help. See all of your help comes from the Lord. God's glory belongs to Him. One thing about it the Lord made you. He made the heavens and the earth.

So, override fear with faith. Take a deep breath and reach for a high call of faith. If you have accepted Jesus as your personal savior then be glad about where you are right now. Focus on where you are now and press toward that mark of a higher calling in Jesus. You can run through troops of attacks that Satan has set for you to trap you, but run on through. (Hebrews 12) Lay aside every weight and sin. So let us strip off and get rid of everything that will hold us back including the sin which is so ready to entangle us, and let us run on through. Let us run with endurance and patience. Let's stay active to the appointed course of the race that is set before us. Run through every troops of disappointment. Run on through.

Problems are going to come on every side when you start out on this journey to walk a holy walk with the Lord. Take one day at a time as you make progress towards the kingdom. The Lord will untie the bound up life that you have carried from generation to generation. He will begin to untie each knot at a time and make you free. All the temptations, persecutions and trials come to run you away from problems, but the Lord says that you are to go through them. Jesus has promised us He will never leave us neither will he forsake us. That's the good news. Child of God run on through.

ATTITUDE CHECK

Keep a good attitude. Bad attitudes hurt our relationships with God and man. First of all get your attitude right with God and it will line up with everyone else. Bad attitudes do hurt our relationships with God.

> Genesis 4:6-7—*So the Lord said to Cain. Why are you angry? And why has your countenance fallen? If you do well, will you not be accepted? And if you do not well sin lies at the door and its desire is for you, but you should rule over it.*

Sometimes we do not offer the lord an act of saving faith. We believe that God exists. We go to worship Sunday morning. We pray on Wednesday nights, but we have the wrong offering, and the wrong attitude. It is almost as if we are saying here we are Lord Take it or leave it. I have learned that obedience is better than sacrifice. Don't just bring anything to the Lord. We know better than anyone on Earth that the Lord loves those whom he chastises. About now we know that we are beings chastised. We may not like it but it is for our good.

Our Father, to you be glory for this dear friend of mine. I ask you to bless this person from the crown of their head to the soles of their feet. If there is sickness, depression, oppression or whatever; Lord heal it in the mighty name of Jesus. Amen

If you keep your head up, keep a good attitude and obey God I believe your blessing of deliverance is on the way. We can have a bad attitude and make some of the worst decisions. Believe me, I have made a few that stagnated me to the point of what seemed to be no return, but you have to believe God if you have been slothful and arrogant. Of course we don't like to wear these titles. We want to call on Jesus. Be glad to have someone who calls it like it is and tells you the truth about yourself. However before you can receive the truth about yourself you have to be able to hear. I am not just talking about our natural hearing. I am speaking of listening with the inner ear. If we do not listen with the inner ear we will not accept the truth.

Let's talk a little more on poor decisions. Being saturated with a bad attitude can cause many terrible situations. It could have caused many of the trials we are going through now. If we had only waited until our thoughts could come from a sound mind and pure heart. We refuse to enter into where God wants us to be. Numbers 14: 1-4 So all the congregation lifted up their voices and cried and the people wept that night and all the children of Israel complained against Moses and Aaron, and the whole congregation said to them, if we had died in the Land of Egypt only if only we had died in this wilderness. Why has the Lord brought us to this land to fall by the sword, that our wives and children should become victims? Would it not be better for us to return to Egypt? So they said to one another, Let us select a leader and return to Egypt.

Poor decisions can lead us back in an Egypt situation, when all God is saying is "trust in me". You have to trust God for your life. When fear grips you like never before this is the time you have to trust God for your life. Nobody can talk about desperate situations like I have seen that involved other people. I have walked through a lot of them myself. My heart goes out to all God's people, and believe me; we are all of His. Some may not confess that they have been saved, but we are all His. For all souls are His. I think some people are more fortunate than others. Some have already learned to trust. When I see programs like Feed the Children and Bishop Jakes on Dr. Phil's show trying to help God's people trust and get back on track. I just honor these people and I hope to meet them one day. To trust God for your life many snares will come but; Proverbs 29:25—The fear of many brings snares, but whoever trust in the Lord shall be safe.

Lord Jesus when I see those big trucks going across the world to carry food to feed your people ; I say one day I am going to be one in the number, because I know favor from you moves mountains. I can do all things through Christ that strengthens me. Amen

Well, we have help, for God will send angels to care for us if we will receive salvation. Hebrews 1:14. This is exciting to know. Angels are spirits sent from God. Of course we do not worship angels. We worship God and when we worship God we are blessed Psalm 24:3-6. The Earth is the Lord's and all its fullness; the world and those who dwell therein. For He has founded it upon the seas, and established it upon the waters. Who may ascend unto the hill of the Lord? Or who may stand in His holy place? He who has cleans hands and a pure heart. He who has not lifted up his soul to an idol nor sworn deceitfully. He shall receive a blessing from the Lord and righteousness from the God of his salvation. This is Jacob, the generation of those who seek Him. Who seek your face. Selah

So have a good attitude, and you should be able now to rejoice, Christians should always rejoice. This does not come overnight or all the time. You grow in grace. It is the grace of God that gives you peace of mind. Satan intended to take you out. We have been stressed from sun op to sun down. The devil is a liar. You have turned another page. The Lord himself has sent his ministering angel to anoint every page. I wish I could explain what I feel right now. I feel the presence of the Lord, and I am blessed. You are going to get your blessing.

BE ANXIOUS FOR NOTHING

Don't be anxious. I had to learn the hard way. I had a sickness called anxiety. This disease almost consumed my life. But God!! Never be anxious. God is working for you while you sleep. Be anxious for nothing, but in everything by prayer and supplication, with thanksgiving let your requests be made known to God. Philippians 4:6

Anxiety is bad stress. I believe we need stress to challenge some issues of life. A little stress causes us to stand up and take charge. When we go through opposition we know that we learn a few things. Don't try to push it away. You certainly can't deny that it is there. If you do not master stress it will master you. When the odds are against you there is triumph in your praise. Psalm 47 O clap your hands, all ye people. Shout unto God with the voice of triumph. For the lord most high is terrible; He is a great king over all the Earth. He shall subdue the people under us, and nations under our feet. He shall choose our inheritance for us, the Excellency of Jacob whom he loved. Selah. God is gone up with a shout, the Lord with the sound of a trumpet. Sing praises to God. Sing praises, sing praises unto our king, Sing praises. For God is the king of all the Earth, Sing ye praises with understanding. God reigneth over the heathen. God sitteth upon the throne of his holiness. The princes of the people are gathered together, even the people of the God of Abraham; for the shields of the Earth belong unto God; He is greatly exalted.

I am moved to say clap your hands and tell the Lord thank you. There are some victories being won right now. When you feel a praise just know you are victorious. When I write about depression, stress and anxiety I realize how blessed I am. I have had many obstacles and challenges in life. My husband of thirty-three years died in 2003 due to kidney failure and other complications. He was a valiant man. He suffered renal failure in his mid to late forties. He was placed on dialysis and remained on dialysis for more than seventeen year. He was fortunate to receive a kidney in 1994. The transplant did work for several years. During his later stages I had to learn how to operate a machine that we could use at home for peritoneal dialysis. It is a very difficult time when you care for people who are sick. It can be very tiresome and depleting. If you are not careful you can become sick yourself. Through it all I count it as a great opportunity. Through this time I relied on help from some well known spiritual giants. I name a few: Bishop Jakes, Ron Parsley, Paula White, Creflo Dollar and Dr. Fred Price. These people offer practical teaching from the Word of God that helps me through these trying times. I believe if I had watched these spiritual giants a little closer I would not have suffered some of the consequences that I experienced.

I have three biological children. They are: Melissa, Esley Jr. and Larnell. Melissa went through some changes during her adolescent years. She did make some mistakes, but I have hope that she will be alright. She is currently incarcerated in a women's correctional facility in the state of Delaware. Melissa had three wonderful children. My first grandchild, Kamekia; the other two are Charles and Santana. I love my grandchildren. I had the opportunity to raise them as my own due to some trying times in my daughter's life. The children needed someone to care for them so I had to be there for them. This seems to be the plight of many grandparents today. They are face with the responsibility of raising their grandchildren. If you are in this situation be encouraged. I will never regret caring for my grandchildren. I had to hang tough through all the crises. When I would read sayings like, Joy comes in the morning time, I reached for joy. Hurt can grip you so it will have you wondering if joy will ever come, but it will.

When Jesus comes into your life; it does not matter about all the things you have been through. You can have joy. You can start having joy right where you are. When God tells you to reach out and help someone, it does not matter if it's your child, a friend or whoever. It is easy to make excuses and keep procrastinating. We intend to obey God. We just say within ourselves that we are going to do it later. Maybe when you feel better or get a better job. You can bless someone with what you have. You may have abundance or just a small amount. Start using what you have. Do not say to your neighbor, go and come again and tomorrow I will give it. Proverbs 3:28

You have to be still and know that God is God. When storms are all around you, you need Jesus to speak in the midst of the storm. We maintain peace by trusting in God. When Jesus and his disciples were crossing the lake and a storm arose the disciples panicked. Sometimes we panic when the storm inside of us is raging. God can speak peace be still. I reached for joy. Hurt can grip you so it will have you wondering if joy will ever come, but it will.

When Jesus comes into your life; it does not matter about all the things you have been through. You can have joy. You can start having joy right where you are. When God tells you to reach out and help someone, it does not matter if it's your child, a friend or whoever. It is easy to make excuses and keep procrastinating. We intend to obey God. We just say within ourselves that we are going to do it later. Maybe when you feel better or get a better job. You can bless someone with what you have.

You have got to take charge right them. It sounds like a lot. We can make it seem greater depending on how we confront the situation. Clean up your act. There is a speedy way out of the storm. All He has to say is peace be still. Tyler Perry is a comic genius. Through his comedies he is able to reach into many lives with life changing truths. It tickles me when I see Meet the Browns. If you are too deep; you cannot not handle them. I love Tyler Perry and all his cast. I would love to meet him someday or maybe even be on a show. Madea mentioned peace be still in one of the plays. I know I am not the only one that had pistol toting ancestors. They would say I am not going to hurt my hand hitting you. I am going to use a piece of steel. My goodness, when we heard those words we lined up, because we thought Queen, my mom, would do just as she said. I have three biological siblings: Josephine, Joseph Ray and Joe Johnson Jr. We can laugh now about all the times of fun and fear we had with our mom and dad. Both of our parents are deceased. I also had the opportunity to care for both of them until I could not give them the care they needed at home. After they were placed in the nursing home I did all I could until they went to be with the Lord. This is another issue in the lives of many people. We have a very large and growing population of elderly citizens. Children are faced with the daunting task of caring for their parents. Through it all God is our present help in time of trouble Psalm 41:1

We would like to think we can do these things on our own. We try but most times we just mess up. Give it over to the Lord right now. Sometimes we have pain from the inside out. I talked about stress being the motivating force in our life that can help push us through. We go through many things in life. We need Jesus to ease the pain. All thing work together for good to those who love God and are called according to His purpose. We can learn a lesson through hurt. Never let it cause you to be bitter, full of hurt and anger. One way to do this is to overcome evil with good by making sure you don't hurt other. Remember all things are working for your good.

God can turn it around for you. You may have had a bad experience. God can turn it around and make it work for you. Sometimes there is a lot of hurt in relationships. Whether it be marriage or friendships. Some of our so called friends can hurt us more than we can bare. You don't have to allow these experiences to destroy your happiness. We can't choose what will happen to us, but we can choose how we respond to it. The way we respond will determine how we will come out. All I can see is you coming out unharmed. I had to pray this prayer so many times. Lord take me thru this and I would love to come out unharmed. I thought about my mind. I wondered I if I would keep my sanity. I was caring for a desperately sick husband. I was also caring for children and grandchildren. We were frequent visitors in hospitals but we made it through by the power of God. Now the children are all grown. All of them graduated high school and some even graduated from college. Some enlisted in the military. My first grandson, Charles Sharon, is a professional football player in the National Football League. We had fun and some real scary times, but we would jump hurdles and keep moving. You keep jumping those hurdles in your life. I feel that you are about to reach your destiny. I feel a prayer in my spirit. It's about 6:30 in the morning and I feel refreshed. Our Father we recognize that only you can help us at this time of crisis. I need your divine guidance to know which way to go. I repent for trying to do what only you can do for me. I ask you for strength for my brothers and sisters and all of the people of God that they will be touched, healed and delivered. In Jesus name. Amen

What a refreshing, your new birth begins in your spirit. You are working with the Holy Spirit to carry out the plan that began to operate in you when you accepted Jesus as you Lord and savior. What I really want to say is remember a chapter or two back in this book when I was going through. Your new birth begins in your spirit which is carried out through your soul which is the mind, will and emotions and then these actions are visible to other people through a manifestation of God's glory on our life. I mean our physical and spiritual life. Amen.

YOU HAVE NOT BEEN LEFT ALONE

Psalm 9:14 Because he has set his love upon me, therefore, will I deliver him. I will set him on high because he has known my name. We have a personal knowledge of his mercy, love, kindness and trust. We rely on him believing he will never forsake us. God wants you to know for a sure thing you are not alone. Satan wants you to believe you are all alone, but you are not. Many believers know and feel what you are going through. As God's child you can claim his wonderful promises regardless of what you are going through. Proclaim that you are not alone as you meditate on God draw strength and encouragement from knowing He may not come when you call Him, but He is always on time. So rejoice because we have this hope that Jesus is Lord.

The Lord of our life, How wonderful it is to know this day right here can be a new beginning of the first day of your life. I am talking about a new start or a fresh start for your life. Every day when we awake that is an opportunity for a fresh start. I come to encourage you that the hero is inside of you. I speak to all ages. Let the potential that is in you come forth into greatness that you never knew was there. You have it, but it needs to come alive.

God wants to bless you and use you for such a time as this. There are lives that need to be touched all over this world. You need to rise up, take a deep breath and just go do it. I don't care what you have been through. Someone else has gone through a greater situation. We call it a catastrophe. We call it a crisis. We have been through some stuff. We kept some of it to ourselves. Just ourselves and God for He knows all things. But when you can tell somebody the Lord knows, you are a life changing phenomenon. That's why it is so important to remember that whatever comes your way "this too shall pass" circumstances, changes, we can remember the good times as well as the bad. They both never last forever. Through Christ that strengthens us we can do all things with joy and peace and show much stability.

Phillipians 4:11 talks about being content. I have learned to be content in other words satisfied to the point I am not disturbed or disgusted in whatever state I am. I find myself rejoicing in times of crisis to the point when it's all over I never knew it could be such a joyful ride. So ride out every storm. What God has for you it is for you. Satan will buffer it out of your mind. So keep your mind on Jesus so that He will keep you in perfect peace.

The Word of God is a therapy. I could stop right here and say a prayer of thanksgiving. Lord the maker of all mankind. The great creator, we give you thanks for being a keeper. You have kept us through some storms that could have taken us out. You did what only you could do. We come to say thank you. These blessings we ask in your son Jesus name. Amen

To the Reader's of this book, this is the beginning of a new day for you. Every page of this book is anointed, but there is a double portion of an anointing that is flowing about now. Take your miracle of healing for your mind, body, soul and spirit and move on to the destiny God has already prepared for you.

Who picked you up?

When I think about the poem, Footprints in the Sand; which I do honor the writer for that. This poem takes us to another level of thoughts. Certainly we did not see or feel the presence of a natural being, but I never could have made it without the help of the Lord. He sustained us from destruction. When weight from every walk of life bashed us down to take us under, Jesus lifted us so high about all of the junk that would have kept us in one place forever, but the mercy of God endures forever and it could not have been nobody but the Lord that picked us ups and turned us around. He took and planted by feet on higher ground. I was sinking deeper and deeper in debt. One evening Jesus picked me up out of a valley of discuss. He showed me that he brought me up out of a dung hill, now rise to another level, even the home you had; you have got to let go and allow me to carry you in the place I have prepared for you. I had to be prepared for what God had for me. Never try to hold on when God calls you to a higher call of praise. Prepare for greatness. Don't be afraid. I must admit I could feel God working shortly after an anointed woman of God prayed for me and prophesied a turnaround would come shortly.

I have not received millions of dollars, but I feel like king's kid. As I sit here at the desk I could write and write. I feel like suddenly I am in a Joyous move. I am on the way to where the Lord is taking me. You also can experience the same exhale and go get your miracle. As is starts your way you can feel a move of, O yes it is real. The presence of the Lord is in your place, your seat, your bathroom working after a glimpse of what God can do. You are more and I mean more than a conqueror because you are a believer. Can you imagine? You can't wait until you tell someone else you have found a man that could tell you everything.

SO MUCH STRENGTH

We are weak, you are strong! 1 Corinthians 4:10, we need help everyday and we need lots of it. Jeremiah 10:23 The way of a man is not in himself. It is impossible for us to run our own life. It does not matter how strong we think we are. It is a mistake to direct our own steps. We cannot properly run our lives until we admit we need the Lord in our lives. This gives us spiritual maturity. I am not saying that we are so weak, but spiritual maturity will take us to another level.

You can take a breath of fresh air and go another mile on your way. Proverbs 18:20 Talking about strength we have an instrument right under our nose that gives us life or death. Can you imagine when we come to acknowledge we have an awesome power right under our nose? Let us use it for the glory of God Proverbs 18:21

Death and life are in the power of the tongue and they who indulge in it shall eat the fruit of it. Let us speak life. You can speak forth—harmony, sickness, disaster, but right now let's speak life into every situation. Take time to thank God Psalm 50: 14-15 Offer to God thanksgiving and pay your vows to the most high. Call upon me in the day of trouble. I will deliver you, and you shall glorify Me.

Let's give thanks unto God, for He alone is worthy of all praise from the rising of the sun to the going down of the same He is worthy to be praised. There is no secret what God can do. Some families have been targeted for years with trials and tribulations, but did not stop because there is hope in the Lord. We have to have a mind to develop our thoughts; because we know what the word of God says what will happen if we put our trust in him. Sometimes taking the first step of faith is hard. I would like to give you some tips of taking steps of faith. All the tips that I am about to five you has helped us all, those that will read this book and receive what the Lord is speaking unto you will do great.

Step one—Look up. I am reminded in the bible days when the psalmist said. I will lift up mine eyes to the hills from whence comes my help. My help comes from the Lord. Even if you fell like your last source of strength is gone hold your head up. Look to the Lord for you help. Step two—Stand up. When you stand up realize that the greater is on the inside of you and you are now walking; you can journey on and when you stand for righteousness, stand for holiness and the Lord will lead you to wherever you need to go.

When you feel discouraged it is sometimes difficult to be positive. That is why you must think about the one who lives in you. Step Three—Rise above. Rise above discouragement. You can do it. The Lord is there for you. He is always available to help you find renewed direction and hope. When I think about how much the Lord cares I want to share it with everyone. So I can meet my many friends face to face. But from this book I can spread the word "Jesus Cares for You".

Jesus will lift you up in due time. His help will come at just the right time. The Word of God says, Humble yourselves, therefore, under God's mighty hand, that He may lift you up in due time. 1Peter 5:6-7 What I really love about the seventh verse is that it says, Cast all your cares, meaning all your anxiety on Him, because He cares for you.

If you have a problem, that is too hard for you to solve, trust the Lord. Just as we roll over on our bed to go to sleep, we never examine the structure to see if it will hold us. We just sit down and roll over. Believe me we cannot do it ourselves. It is an awesome thing to know, we have a savior, whose thoughts are not our thoughts his ways are not our ways, praise God.

I have three biological children: Melissa, Esley & Larnell. They all are hard workers of course. Melissa is going through a trying time; I believe some of what inspired me to write this book. I had to exhale. To bare the things Melissa went through, she is now at Baylor correctional Institute for Women. She is serving time for a crime that Satan himself inflicted on her. She has been there for about five years. With the help of God, her brothers, we have managed to survive this far. Melissa is my only daughter. I brag on her all the time. I do not know the situation, but a struggle ensued and Melissa was spared. I am very sorry for the other person that lost his life. Melissa was charged with first degree manslaughter in the state of Delaware. Her life has changed tremendously and I believe she is going to be alright. For God has a way that we will not understand until it is all over. There is so much greatness for her. I miss her from being outside the walls, but she continues to trust God. There is a destiny for her; she will be able to tell somebody how she made it over. Thank God.

Esley and Larnell are my heroes. They along with Melissa served as a companion and friend to my very sick husband, who has gone to be with the Lord.

That's a little story about the kids. They are all great helpers. That's why I can say I miss Melissa. She was my right hand lady. So we must hang tough.

Every time I think of how Jesus was led into the wilderness to be tested, and tried by the devil. He did not complain or become discouraged and depressed. He went through each test victoriously. Can you imagine Jesus complaining? You and I have the mind of Christ and love the thought. We can handle things the way He did for the joy of the Lord is our strength. Experience is the greatest teacher. When you go through you can tell someone else they can make it. So by being mentally prepared through victorious thinking, we will make it to our destiny. So much strength will come alive in you. You will find strength to get up out of your comfort zone. Oh yes you are in the zone now. The majority of people already have some abilities in them. It is amazing what can come from the inside out, a master builder, an attorney, a secretary, an accountant; you name it. If you ever come to reality, EXHALE! And say I am going to do whatever it takes to reach the goals I have set.

TRUST AND REJOICE

You must give a listening ear to what the Lord is saying about your situation. He may be saying "stand still", but you are moving to the left and to the right and trying to fix things yourself.

Never give up is my motto. I have heard different ones say you can't just sit down and do anything to help yourself. Get up and do something. It is amazing to know how educated and talented you are. Until you get up and use that intellectual ability you will never prove what's on the inside of you. A chap always goes to the finish line. I don't care how things may seem you will get there. Your destiny is not too far ahead, so keep moving. Trust me, we all need some guidelines. God's word is a good way to prepare you for the battle. Set some goals. What are your plans? Believe me; every plan begins with a desire, a goal or a dream. Now it's okay to have an earthly mentor; someone that will be available to help you. Your mentor will tell you the truth. Sometimes we just don't want to hear that, but the harder the bump on a natural road, soon you will see the traveling gets easier and easier. You will soon be a winner. I believe you are about to do a complete turnaround and head in the right direction. Why? Because you trust God. Amen.

LOVE YOU

Mornings are special, because it is the dawn of a new day. Fresh air meets you head on, especially when you take time to go for a walk. I encourage you to walk shortly after sunrise. You will get a double dose. Unless you are medically restricted I believe a little sun shine is good. Love you. If you don't have a walking partner you just go out there and walk and breathe in the fresh air. Love yourself so much that you include a little encouragement from yourself. Say to yourself today I will encourage myself. As you read this section on love you might be going through a crisis of sickness in your body. Some time we just neglect to go the things we need to do to have a healthier, happier life. All we need to do is love ourselves.

To be or not to be motivated; that is the question. We need to be motivated in order to go places. We must take responsibility to meet every need that we have. Believe me we can't get everything done to satisfy ourselves. Sometimes we can't satisfy our wants even for one day. But be grateful for the fact you are not procrastinating, but you have sparked a new look on life.

I wrote this book because of a spark. I felt inspired to share testimonies of what God can do. I joy and I write because I believe whoever comes in contact with these writing will rejoice. When things are created they come with an instruction manual. Your manufacturer has given you the instructions on how to operate and get your troublesome problem fixed.

I find that in the word of God, God has set a plan, which is the laws and believe me it really works. This law is called the Holy Bible for my mind, body, soul and spirit. It is the best manual in the world. A God sent manual from the great creator, the Lord God almighty. You will love this, because you will feel better about yourself. Obedience to the word of God will produce the best results for a healthy, happy and righteous life for you. Eat right, exercise and get an adequate amount of sleep daily. Take good care of yourself. This is a primary priority. You owe this to yourself. Through different time of sickness I been advised to drink a sufficient amount of water; it works.

Isaiah 12:1

And in that day thou shalt say, O Lord I will praise thee though thou wast angry with me, thine anger is turned away and thou comfortedst me

2 Behold, God of salvation; I will trust and not be afraid. For the Lord JEHOVAH is my strength and my song he also is become my salvation.3 Therefore with joy shall ye draw water out of the wells of salvation.

Our father we thank you for guidance. Today we receive your instructions for a better life spiritually, physically and financially. For your hand is not shortened that it cannot reach down and save. For it was you that brought us from the midst of destruction. Thank you Lord. Amen

LAY YOUR WORRIES DOWN

God has promised us in his word that he would never leave us neither would he forsake us. When we stop right now and consider what is worrying you; Remember God is a praying hearing, promise keeping, forgiving God. Never too late, but he is always on time. Some have said, and I to believe, He may not come when you want him, but he is on time. When we realize that God's law is forever, our little worries will diminish. Be comforted that he has everything under control.

Father I lay aside every sin and worry that is going to keep me from running to you. For I long to learn your statues which you have established forever. Yearning for God caused a leap of faith

Psalm 42:1

As the deer pants for the water brooks so pants my soul for you, O God my soul thirst for God, for the living God. When shall I come and appear before God.

Your very soul can thirst for God not only will you seek one time, but you will keep on searching for the living God. I can visualize the deer searching until it finds what it needs. The deer search for the brook, a time of refreshing. God is peace in the midst of distress. Praise our God.

TIME OUT

When educators see this phrase they can relate. Everyone knows the purpose of a time-out. Now I don't mean time out on the town; going out to dinner or shopping. I am speaking of some time to think about where you come from and where you are now.

Remember some parents have struggles much different from others, but all of us have to take time to think. We should ask the question, where should we go from here? While we are spending time thinking; Let us appreciate the power of be educated through the power of God. The hands that formed us are the same hands that teach us. Lord give us understanding to learn your commands.

According to Psalm 119:73-80

Your hands made me and formed me. Give me understanding to learn your commands. God is concerned about our physical needs as well as our spiritual needs, so here we can see the power of being educated. We need to take time out to listen to what the leading of the Holy Spirit is saying to us. The Lord who made us helps us to learn. We need to focus on him for he was the inventor of a great lesson plan from the beginning.

> *Our Father we realize how great you are thank you for teaching us the way through your holy word.*

A MAJOR BREAKTHROUGH

When you go to the next level it is like a mountain climber who seeks to go a little higher than the place that he or she stood at a particular time. We need to persevere like a mountain climber. We can make it through crisis and circumstances by praying and believing in yourself. Having confidence in you and the things you can do will cause your whole family to reap benefits. I know that many are apprehensive because of the economy. Many families need to consider where they are now and where they would like to go. We need to remember the teachings of our grandparents. Granny taught is how to cut back. She taught us how wait on things we might not need right now. We can get through by helping each other. I am sure you have some thoughts that you could reach back and give a helpful hint to help somebody. When I started to write this book I had no idea we would go through an economic recession. As a matter of fact this is an experience for me. Perhaps the last recession I probably was a child a home. I could not understand why we could not have the things we would like to have.

My grandmother, Lizzie Hicks Jones, raised me. I loved her so much. She was a courageous woman. She was a woman who had a high moral standard for living. I watched her do a lot of great things like gardening and caring for livestock. I have recollections of my friend, Dot, and me chasing chickens and having so much fun. We would run the chickens out of there nesting places and make play houses.

Have you ever sensed a move of God and then something great just happened? Well I feel like there is a major breakthrough that is about to happen. We can pray that the economy will get better. Only good common sense can work for such a time as this. Don't worry; one of my helpful points from God's word is to put your trust in the Lord. With the hand of God applied together with these times and situations that seem to be out of control; we are going to make it. Rejoice even when it seems like nothing is moving, nothing is happening for you, all the time something great is happening. O yes and it is working for your good. Sometimes we need to exhale and ask the Lord to help us. The majority of the time the blessing we need is just a prayer away. I remember seven years ago, an evangelist came to town; I was doing through some difficult times. The evangelist told me your blessing is just a prayer away, but instead of me trusting and not doubting the word, that she said, until one day I thought a prayer away could be the very next time I go to God in prayer. Well it happened. Never in a lifetime did I think It would happen the way I least expected, but believe me I got a breakthrough. Some release came out of nowhere. I want to say to you yes you are next in line for a miracle. Learn to pray for yourself.

Seven steps that will motivate you to get up.

1. Time waits on no one
2. Discern what Satan is doing to you.
3. Realize the authority in you.
4. Come clean with yourself.
5. Confess that you need help.
6. Someone needs your testimony.
7. If the Lord said it that settles it.

> *Our Father, I pray for my friends today. Wherever they are; I ask you to reveal the truth in every part of their life. Lord you are revealing the healing and deliverance experience like I have received and I fell right now you are doing great and wonderful things in their life because your presence is here. Lord we are hungry and thirsty for righteousness. We ask you to purify our minds, sanctify our hearts and let your ministering angels encamp round about us and protect us so we will never fall into the pitfalls of Satan. Lord make the word come alive in us that we might be able to jump every hurdle. We give you the praise. Help us to conquer and destroy carnality that we might be able to see and hear what the Holy Spirit is saying to us. I ask all these blessing in the name of Jesus. Amen*

The gospel is being preached all over the world. We have hope. What I love about it is the bible is right all by itself. If I were you, my friend, and had not confessed that Christ has come in your life; I would repent and receive the Lord in my life today. Don't put off today for tomorrow. While you have this great opportunity; do it now. You will say like the psalmist said "O how I love thy law! It is my meditation all the day Psalm 119: 97

The value of diligence is staring you in your face daily, so do what is coming to your mind today, the things that benefit you in the future. Go back to college and finish this time. Start a business. Help someone to know it is not over until God says it is over.

SOMEONE NEEDS YOUR TESTIMONY

For the ear test words as the palate taste food. Let us choose what is right let us determine among ourselves what is good. We become well balanced, vigilant and cautious at all times because we realize the enemy is as a roaring lion seeking whom he may devour. IPeter 5:8.

Take a few encouraging words from a friend. You do not have to run anymore child of God. You have authority to defeat him in the name of Jesus. At the latter part of an illness, Satan came to attack my mind, will and emotions. I could not work on a steady job or face traffic on a highway. I was sick with anxiety, but exercising authority over the enemy, speaking a word of faith over my situation; I have victory in the Lord. When I think about pressing toward the mark of a higher calling I get joy down in my soul! The joy of the Lord is my strength.

You say you got Jesus? If you confess Jesus Christ as your personal savior, you have authority over the enemy. You are blessed because you trust in the Lord. Jeremiah 17:8 says They shall be like a tree planted by the water. Can you imagine standing against the enemy? Know that the Lord is with you. You don't have to worry. The Greater One is on the inside.

Admit that you are not perfect, and I must say we are not. But according to Roman 3:23 for we all have sinned and come short of the glory of God. Self help is the greatest source you can have. You know you are experiencing some difficult situations! Sometimes we will not confess.

But thank God for grace and mercy, sometimes I believe mercy runs us down. Mercy goes before all of us helping us, our children and our families. It also helps our neighbors and friends. Grace and mercy is there to satisfy any problem. Free yourself for help is on the way. Trust in the Lord's unfailing love. Psalm 13:5-6

Even the greatest athlete needs help sometimes. The greatest doctor need more than just a tool in the emergency room or operating room, but they need to confess that they need help. Prayer is the key and we want to keep our thoughts faith based. Sometimes we can't connect with anyone else but God. Although it is a good thing to have someone to rescue us when we need help we must do the things that we need to do. The Lord is here he will come into you. Just open your mouth and let the Holy Ghost use you to tell him Lord send me some help. I do believe help will be on the way.

Some of us have run well. Keep running in a spiritual race. The Lord is with you. You have fought a good fight. You have kept the faith. When it gets really bad, crisis happens, keep holding on. Be patient. You have run well, you talked about what God has brought you through and believe me somebody heard the word. They ask God and seek him. I feel the Holy Ghost as I get ready to close this chapter for the steps for motivation to get you up and going. People of God men will be going and women will be glowing. Boys and girls will be richly clothed in joy because they trusted the word of God.

I Timothy 6:12 fight the good fight of faith. Lay hold on eternal life whereunto thou art also called and had professed a good profession before many witnesses. Praise the Lord!

Don't be a stranger, when it comes time to tell of his goodness. It is alright to tell how the Lord brought you and you know you didn't do it yourself.

I get a chance to do ministry at a local correctional facility. I get joy in telling the inmates that God has allowed them to be there. I tell them of the situations in which I have been involved. I know that it was the mercy of God that keeps us alive because we all could have been destroyed trying to get away from the police or challenging someone. Many times we did not even know what we were so angry about. We just didn't have Christ in our lives. Child of God you are blessed. Tell of his goodness. Sometimes what seems like nothing to us means much to another person. If you have been in situation that seem like you were just going to die you might have been told by a doctor that you can't be healed, but a miracle came out of nowhere. You might have escaped a terrible accident. I know I did. I escaped a tractor and trailer accident. It hit my PT cruiser and the voice of an angel spoke to me. It said ride it out or die. By moving speedily I was blessed to come out wonderfully unharmed with a scratch on my car the width of a fingernail. Glory to God!

The greatness in you will come forth and spark a flame of concern in the life of someone else. Please read this book and tell someone else that it had to be the Lord that has brought you this far. There is Destiny for you. I believe you are destined to be great. Since we are talking about destiny your walk in the Word will keep you in good working order. There are operator and trouble shooters on standby 24-7 to walk us through difficult situations. We are likely to call a family member or friend, but if you think about it somewhere around the house you have a manual that will fix any problem. The manual is the Word of God.

AUTHOR'S BIOGRAPHY

Prophetess Rebecca Boykin is a native of the great Sunshine State, Florida. I was born in Palatka Fl to the late Queen Ivy Jones and Ernest Starling. I was raised by the most honorable stepfather one could find. His name was Joe Johnson Sr. The union of Queen Ivy Jones and Joe Johnson produced some of the finest siblings in the world. They are Josephine, Joseph Ray and Joe Johnson Jr. I also have other sibling through the lineage of Earl Starling. I have a lot of precious memories about my upbringing. I fondly remember the hot sand piles in our back yard, because we did not have grass in some areas. I would walk on my heels until I made it through the sand to our back porch.

I accepted the Lord, Jesus Christ, as my savior at the age of 23. I love every bit of my saved life. The salvation that Jesus offers make one has compassion for people. I love to see everyone happy.

I have been a member of Holy Temple of God Incorporated. I served faithfully under the bishopric of the late Bishop Walter Camps Sr. for approximately 30 years. I have also served under Dr. Mamie Bryant in our home church in East Palatka, FL for almost four decades. I am the founder and president of the organization's Women's Auxiliary. The Lord called me into the prophetic realm over 20 years ago. The most joyous part of my life is to know that I have had an impact on someone's life.

I love to see people survive whatever they go through; you can make it! I want to speak to families around the world. Parents you can be a star for your family with the Lord being the head of your life. Sometimes we say the Lord is the head of our life; but, is he really the head of our life? Do we pray and ask for his guidance before we get into troublesome times?, Absolutely not. We'll try to fix it ourselves. Never forget how you were through one crisis after another. You have to hold out and learn the strategies of the devil. Remember it is not our children; It is the enemy which is the devil working to destroy them.

We need to be like track runners. The Lord lets us lay aside every weigh and sin that would so easily beset us. Let us run with patience. The word of God is great.

Sometime or another you are going to be able to lift up your hands and rejoice; why, because a release has come in your household. Speaking of households; I would love to speak a word of prayer over your family right now.

Our father, we bless your holy name. I ask you today to stretch out your hand of deliverance as I touch and agree with the person who has come into contact with this website. Father we ask these blessings in Jesus name Amen.

Prayer changes things

Let's talk about keeping our natural body healthy, we have talked about our soul, Lay aside weights and sin. Well that is the spiritual side of us. It is very important to maintain good health. This is really what my book is all about. You don't need to carry baggage. Carrying baggage is too much for you. A good smile; I believe is a health factor. I believe it helps the circulation if blood. I am not a doctor, but I believe your smile means so much to that person you meet whether it is in your home, church or neighborhood grocery store. Sometimes we just need a smile.

So in the run of a day let go. Exhale a breath of fresh air and release the things you have been holding. It can be a small thing that you think can do no harm. Get rid of it. You are not on the track field anymore. Let's get real. You don't have natural weights on your ankle. I am talking about your attitude. Do an attitude check. Daily ask yourself, am I looking holy, but doing things I am not supposed to? Am I mean to other people? Do I hold grudges against other? Love is what is going to lift you out of this.

Exercising the love of God to the spiritual body will cause the natural body to line up. I believe we can overcome a lot of sickness with the right attitude. As I have stated, you are going to be so blessed to be able to clean your closet, rearranged yourself, get out there and doing something for yourself. A new you will arrive on the scene.

Go forth, you can make a change. When a change comes over you your neighbor might not recognize who you are; you will be looking so good. God has a way of renewing your strength. He will bring you out. I don't care what you have been through. God is able to carry you through.

Get up now. I am about to close with tears almost welling up in my eyes. I am rejoicing for you. Praise God for you. Men, women, boys&girls it's yours. I am so impressed with 'Exhale for the Lord our God is With Thee. It embodies the principles to help you focus on what God can do in your life.

Rebecca Boykin—A prophetess, exhorter, author, motivational speaker and prophetic mime

The Author, Rebecca Boykin, shares crisis and testimonies of the overcoming power of the hand of God. Many people have been saved and set free from strongholds that they never thought they could be freed from.